Please Doctor, I'd Rather Do It Myself... with Vitamins and Minerals!

LaDean Griffin

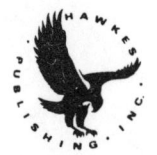

Published by
HAWKES PUBLISHING, INC.

3775 South 500 West
Salt Lake City, Utah 84115
Tel. (801) 262-5555

© Copyright 1979

Hawkes Publishing, Inc.

ISBN 0-89036-120-7

Printed in the U.S.A.

Illustrations & Cover by
Rod Warren

TABLE OF CONTENTS

Preface... 13

Introduction 14

VITAMINS 24

    A 24

    B Complex 27

    B1 30

    B2 33

    B6 36

    B12 39

    B Factors

        Biotin 42

        Choline.................................... 43

        Folic Acid 46

        Inositol 48

        Niacin, B3................................ 50

        Pantothenic Acid 52

        PABA..................................... 55

    Panganic Acid 57

    Vitamin C 59

    Vitamin D 64

    Vitamin E 66

    Vitamin F 69

    Vitamin K 70

    Vitamin P 72

MINERALS 75

    Calcium 75

    Chromium 78

    Cobalt 79

    Copper 80

    Iodine 82

    Iron 84

    Magnesium 87

    Manganese 90

    Phosphorus 92

    Potassium 94

Silicon 99

Sodium.................................... 100

Sulphur................................... 103

Zinc...................................... 105

VITAMIN AND MINERAL DEFICIENCIES AND DISEASES............................ 108

Acne 108

Alcoholism 108

Allergies 108

Anemia 108

Appetite Loss 109

Arteriosclerosis 109

Arthritis 109

Aspirin Poisoning........................ 109

Baldness 109

Barbiturate Overdose 110

Black Widow Spider Bites 110

Bleeding Gums 110

Blood Clots 110

Broken Bones 110

Bruises 110

Burns 110

Carbon Monoxide Poisoning 110

Cataracts 111

Cirrhosis 111

Cold Hands & Feet 111

Colds 111

Colitis 111

Constipation 111

Dandruff 111

Dehydration 111

Depression 111

Dermatitis 111

Detached Retina 112

Diabetes 112

Diarrhea 112

Digestive Disorders 112

Disc Troubles 112

Dizziness 112

Dry Skin 112

Eczema 112

Emphysema 112

Encephalitis 113

Fatigue 113

Fever 113

Frostbite 113

Gallstone 113

Goiter 113

Gray Hair 113

Hair Color Restored......................... 113

Halitosis 113

Hay Fever................................... 113

Headache.................................... 113

Heart Disease 114

Heatstroke 114

Hemorrhage.................................. 114

Hernia 114

Insomnia 114

Joint Troubles 114

Kidney Infection 114

Kidney Stones 114

Leg Cramps 114

Liver Problems 114

Loss of Taste 115

Meningitis................................. 115

Menopause 115

Menstrual Cramps 115

Menstrual Problems 115

Mental Illness 115

Mental Retardation 115

Migraine Headache 115

Miscarriage 115

Motion Sickness 115

Mouth Sores 115

Muscular Disorders 115

Nausea 116

Nervousness 116

Neuralgia 116

Night Vision............................... 116

Overactive Thyroid 116

Overweight................................. 116

Pain....................................... 116

Parasitic Disease 116

Phlebitis 116

Poison Oak or Ivy 116

Poisonous Bites 117

Polio 117

Poor Circulation 117

Premature Aging 117

Prostate Troubles 117

Psoriasis 117

Psychosis 117

Radiation Poison 117

Respiratory Flu............................ 117

Retarded Growth 117

Rheumatic Fever 117

Rheumatism 118

Rocky Mtn. Spotted Fever 118

Sciatica 118

Senility 118

Sensitivity to Light or Sun 118

Shortness of Breath 118

Sinusitis 118

Skin Spots 118

Slight Paralysis 118

Sore Throat, Strep 118

Sterility 118

Stomach Ulcers 119

Stress 119

Sunburn 119

Swollen Glands 119

Tooth Decay 119

Ulcers 119

Virus Diseases 119

Voice Box Gives Out Easily 119
Wrinkles 119

PREFACE

How many times has your family felt sick in some way and rushed off to the doctor? He then suggests a list of drugs for you to take. By the time the doctor and pharmacists are through, the strain on your pocket book has made you even more ill. The drugs fail to do their job, make you drowsy, and often cause other side effects to your system. You are left to wonder if there isn't another way?

There is another way: In so many instances you can heal yourself with the proper selection of vitamins and minerals!

With this beautiful book, you can learn the daily doses of vitamins and minerals needed to improve your health; foods that can destroy certain vitamins; nutrients that will augment each vitamin; and the food sources for each vitamin. Name your illness or condition and you will find a vitamin that will improve your health.

When you get through with this book, you will be excited about vitamins and minerals and you will be confident in feeling you now know how to be healthier and happier without the doctor and drugs.

You will discover more Vim, Vigor, and Vitality from Vitamins and Minerals!

INTRODUCTION

A 'vitamin from natural sources' generally means a concentrated food rich in a particular vitamin — with fat, moisture and fibers removed. Other factors in the concentrate the biochemists call 'impurities', such things as the unknowns, the trace minerals, amino acids, enzymes, etc.

Occasionally the FDA will insist that certain known factors be excluded from supplements just because they are unproven. Because of this unresolved scientific dispute some known factors are excluded on these grounds alone. These known and unknown factors remain and exist in a more natural concentrate. If some of these factors are non-essential to you as they occur in nature, which is doubtful, you have nothing to lose. However, if they are essential, even though their function is yet unknown, it could possibly be critical to you.

The word *natural* has been used and abused until, like the word *organic*, much confusion exists as to the correct usage of the word. A definition of 'natural' in its use here would be as they occur in nature naturally with both known and unknown factors existing, while a 'synthetic' is created in the laboratory from so-called organic or inorganic

Introduction

substances unrelated to the foods in which the vitamins being produced would naturally occur. (a *crystalline* starts out as a natural and goes through a series of solvents until only the pure, isolated vitamin with none of the so-called impurities remain in crystalline form).

The word *organic* has been much abused also from what the original organic gardner intended. Anything containing the carbon molecule today is considered organic, even coal or petroleum. The fact, however, that the words 'natural' and 'organic' have been much used and abused still leads everyone to believe that such things are becoming more and more important. It may even suggest that the scientists who have said there is no difference between organic and inorganic, synthetic or natural, are losing ground. What really counts in the long run is how such organic or inorganic, synthetic or natural, feels in the human body.

Cake, cigaretts, alcohol, coffee and candy didn't get the reputation for being unhealthy merely because someone said so. If a person says he does not smoke or drink, the other person will usually say, "Oh, you don't have any bad habits." Who told him they were bad habits? Why don't mothers and fathers give their babies coffee to drink for breakfast? Why do we keep a limit on the age to smoke and drink? How do people know these things are bad? Because of how it feels in the human body.

We don't need any scientist to tell us so. If this is true, then it naturally follows that how the vitamins feel in the body is what counts, not what a scientist supposes it should do.

On a recent talk show a medical doctor called in to challenge me. He stated that more scientific research and blind studies needed to be done on herbs. My answer to him was that through the drug use and abuse period of the past 50 years or so, there had always been the counter culture of people who used herbs, vitamins and natural food. They have known how to combat and prevent disease and have known how it feels in the body to obey nature's rules, and somehow they didn't feel it was necessary to prove it to the world, even though they had proven it to themselves. He continued to challenge me, so my argument was: so what if science finds out what poisons me in a drug? How many ways can it hurt me for the few things it does? It does not seem logical to me to use such a dangerous substance, when I know how well I can feel with natural elements.

People who use natural vitamins and get results are not intimidated by illogical scientific argument. The people who have been really sick and have run the gauntlet of the drug method and somehow found their way to natural foods, natural vitamins and herbs, are the ones who do most proselyting for a healthier way because they have been there. They know first-hand the difference in how their bodies feel with one method or the other.

American citizens of today can boast 100 million cases of chronic disabling diseases. This is nearly half of the population, and the other half works to support them. One in every 16 Americans aches with arthritis and rheumatism, not to mention the 250,000 children afflicted with arthritis. Every year more than a million people die of vascular disease. 97% of Americans have some kind of chronic dental disease. Who are we kidding with longevity statistics? There is a lot to be said for living while you are alive, and not living most of your life half dead.

Statistics lull us away into a false security because we are a rich nation, both in food and materials. We can afford to be charitable now, but what about hard times or famine with insufficient resources to maintain the institutions which house such people and pay welfare and disability payments? Could these statistics change under these circumstances? If American righteousness has kept up with its wealth, perhaps we could still be a charitable people. History does not convince us, however, that righteousness and wealth walk hand in hand. We are a sick nation. Autopsies performed on soldiers during the Korean war, with the average age of 22 years, revealed some degree of arteriosclerosis in over three-fourths of the cases. In

12% of these, arterial obstruction exceeded the 50% level — and this group was considered the best young people we had.

When America has the highest rate of infection per capita of any society, even higher than India, with all our sanitation practices, antibiotics and so-called 'pharmaceutical advances', we need to take a long, hard look at how we feel; not what science keeps trying to persuade us to believe.

Many years ago my uncle, who was a horticulturist, ran his own private test when the new chemical fertilizers first came on the market. Taking two tomato plants and planting them side by side, with one stake between them on which they could both climb, having prepared the soil on the one side with chemical fertilizer and the other with organic matter compost, he began his vigil to see just what would happen. The plants began to grow, climbing the stake together, intertwining with one another. As they grew larger, he began to observe the difference in vigor, beauty and health of the organically composted plant. He noticed aphids beginning to come onto the plant feeding on the chemical ground. Strange how it didn't affect the stronger organic plant. What could he do to save the sick plant? The only thing he could have done — and this is the answer people find today — spray it with poison to kill the bugs. Does this tell you anything?

Introduction

The chemical companies have gradually become an enormous business. The arguments have vascillated between organic people and the chemical companies. The one thing that chemical growers could never argue with was taste and flavor — organic tastes better. Organic people claimed that people living on organic food were healthier because the food they were eating was healthier. The chemical farmer claimed that they could also grow food as large or larger and just as beautiful as anything grown with compost. Their biggest and best argument is, "Who could feed the world population on organically composted foods? It is too time consuming, so leave us alone. We are at least getting the job done, providing for the world's peoples."

There has now developed a bridge between these two factions — a compromise that will eventually bless the world's people. Let me begin at the beginning. The balance of minerals has been so upset that it borders on insanity. It has gone so far it would take years to repair the situation, even with organic composting methods. Society cannot wait that long. Foods grown from depleted soil cannot be expected to be mineral rich.

We have made great strides in biological science that can presumably identify genes which cause learning disabilities. We have had so many brain-damaged and birth-defected children that our institutions are full to capacity. We spend an enormous amount of money each year to try to rehabilitate such children. Now the cry is that we need to stop producing such children. Thus, a mother can easily have a child aborted if she feels she cannot cope with such a disability.

We have coined two new words — *brain dysfunction* for the slow learning child and *hyperactive* or *hyperkenetic* for the too-busy-to-learn child. School systems, science and parents have decided that the way to control the learning for these types of children is to drug them. They are given speed or downers, like the illicit drugs found on the streets. Everyone seems to be concerned with the learning disability or acceptable behavior, but when a child is a nuisance or a menace, no one seems to be concerned with the child's silent agony. There have been no proofs as to the child's improved ability to learn by these methods. All that has been accomplished is to calm the hyperactive child so that the teacher and parent can stand them or salve the conscience of those who deal with the brain-dysfunctioned, into believing they are doing something for these behavioral misfits. The so-called technology to put a child in such a slot is so weak in its diagnosis and treatment, its masked secrecy only tends to enhance the mystical powers ascribed to the tester.

When will we learn to feed our children the necessary vitamins and minerals through good, live, whole foods from rich soil to solve these problems? America's sugar consumption is up to almost 150 lbs. per person per year. It was said several years ago that by 1980 one in five would be diabetic. The world, especially America, is drunk with sugar, not to mention all the other junk food. Our future generations will pay the price of our folly. We give our children baskets full of sugar for Easter, treats for Halloween, birthday cakes, candy for Christmas. Sugar is in almost every food that is put on the table.

The latest thing in agriculture today may be the saving factor: vegetation from the sea for mineral supplements and sea water for the plants instead of chemical fertilizers. Since all the ground has been so depleted that many of those who have argued that they can produce just as good a food as organic gardeners are realizing that they have been mistaken. They have done a similar thing as the drug people have done.

Drugs do something in the body, it is certain; but they often work like whipping a tired horse, as with cortisone, until the gland is burned out, or they leave a residue that later becomes chronic disease like the tomato plant full of germs and parasites. The reason for this is because man was never intended to live on a mono-diet. All the foods that grow are widely spread with the minerals and vitamins he requires. He was never intended to eat the dirt or the rock, which is definition for 'inorganic.' Yet he fills his body with drugs made from potash rock and petroleum — inorganic by such standards, made from coal and salts from rock. When he uses all of these inorganic substances he is still much different from the plant who eats dirt or rock to grow, and doesn't care if it is chemical. If all the plant substances were broken down, as in compost, to become usable fuel for the plant, this would be nature's way and the best way.

The chemical fertilizer growers could have grown almost as well as the organic farmer if he had put in all the minerals. Since they are many unknowns in the vitamin business, how could he accomplish this? He made the big mistake of putting only three major chemicals in the ground. These three are phosphorus, nitrates and potash. Potash may have contained some unknowns and extras, but most plants require 44 known minerals to be healthy. Some can get by with 35. Lettuce growers know they need an alkiline soil, and zinnia growers know it must be acid.

The complex structures of plants must build on these 35 to 44 minerals to produce their own vitamins. When this cannot be achieved the plant becomes diseased. What the chemical fertilizer people did not realize was that by stimulating the growth with the major minerals they used, the plant would have to leach the soil to match the amounts so as to cause this greater growth demand created. This results in an eventual deficiency in the soil. When the soil has no natural replacements to build it up, this creates disease, the need for poison spray and also tasteless foods are created. What happens to people who live on such depleted food?

Now the bridge has been found between the organic gardener and the chemical fertilizer companies. Most companies are looking into the possibility of replacing the nutrients with sea water. This may save us for a while, but there is still the need for whole vegetation replacement back into the soil. In the meantime, wiser people realize the need for a good food supplement. This must be achieved in the only real place left on earth to find such essential nutrients — the sea and nature's wild, untouched, uncultivated places. These healthful vitamins and minerals must be made with a base of sea vegetation and nature's wild uncultivated herbs.

SECTION I
VITAMINS

MDA was used as a standard of average minimum or very smallest daily requirements to prevent deficiency. United States Recommended Daily Allowances, or RDA, means a standard set by the food & drug administration. This standard has never been established as the complete fulfillment of nutritional requirements. Many nutrients have not been officially established. IU means international units and is used as a measure for Vitamins A, D, & E.

VITAMIN A
        Daily dose — RDA — 5,000 IU
        Approx. restore — 10,000 - 25,000 IU
        Toxicity — 50,000 IU

Destroyed by:

        alcohol
        coffee
        cortisone
        excessive iron
        mineral oil
        Vitamin D deficiency

Part of the Body Essential For:

        eyes
        bones

hair
soft tissue
teeth
lungs

Symptoms of Deficiency:

night blindness
impaired vision
difficulty to adapt to darkness
glued eyelids
skin troubles (acne, boils, impetigo)
dandruff
brittle nails & hair
loss of hearing
loss of taste & smell
stone formations
psoriasis
warts
wrinkles
gallstones
liver problems
red eyelids
bone or joint pain
itchy, burning eyes
dry mouth
unable to store fat
dry lips
hair loss
dry genitourinary system
vitamin A poisoning

Nutrients which Augment:

    B Complex
    Choline
    Vitamins C, D, E
    Calcium
    Phosphorus
    Zinc

Foods & Sources:

    (small amounts in all foods)
    watermelon
    raw carrot juice
    yellow & green foods
    alfalfa
    dandelion
    lambsquarter
    okra pods
    paprika
    cayenne
    grape leaves
    red raspberries
    violet
    butter fat
    kale
    cabbage
    (a sprig of parsley contains as much
      Vita. A as a glass of raw carrot juice)
    fish liver oils
    milk fat
    apricots-dried (3 apricots = 3,000 IU
    1 peach = 1,330 IU

½ cantalope = 9,240 IU
liver-beef — ½ lb. = 50,000 IU
spinach = 8,000 IU
carrots — raw - 1 med. = 10,000 IU

Useful For:
body tissues repaired & maintained
resists infection
night vision

The liver stores excess of Vitamin A, allowing it to be released as needed. Some conditions of the body such as liver disease and infections prohibit absorption of Vitamin A.

Mineral oil, when taken internally, carries away Vitamin A so it cannot be absorbed.

Higher doses are required during pregnancy & lactation — 6,000 - 8,000 IU.

Malnourishment or serious trauma are good reasons for high restoration doses of Vitamin A.

Vitamin A fights infection.

VITAMIN B COMPLEX (Water soluble)
Daily dose — RDS — See B Vitamins
Approx. restore — See B Vitamins

Destroyed By:

 birth control pills
 coffee
 stress
 sugar
 sulpha drugs
 sleeping pills
 infections
 alcohol

Part of the Body Essential For:

 eyes
 gastrointestinal tract
 hair
 liver
 mouth
 brain
 ears
 soft tissue
 muscles
 blood
 energy
 metabolism of carbohydrates fat & protein
 muscle tone

Symptoms of Deficiency:

 acne
 anemia
 constipation
 high cholesterol

Vitamins

    digestive problems
    fatigue
    hair (dull, falling out, dry)
    dry skin
    rough skin
    insomnia

Nutrients which Augment:

    Vitamin C
    Calcium
    Vitamin E
    Phosphorus

Foods & Sources:

barley	almonds
bananas	brazil nuts
figs	coconut
strawberries	haddock
watermelon	poultry
rutabagas	ice cream
veal	honey
asparagus	molasses
brussel sprouts	yeast
carrots	alfalfa
cauliflower	artichokes
lettuce	beans
cabbage	soy beans
celery	broccoli
cucumbers	okra
lentils	parsley
leeks	peanuts
mushrooms	parsnips

peas
peppers
sauerkraut
wheat
rye
avocados
cantaloupe
peaches
yogurt

potatoes
tomatoes
turnips
corn
apples
dates
oranges
raisins

Useful For:

alcoholics
allergies
baldness
heart abnormalities
hyperglycemia
migraine headaches
menstrual difficulties
hyperactive children

psychosis
anemia
barbituate
overdose
cystitis
stress
overweight

VITAMIN B1 (Thiamin) (Water soluble)

Daily dose — RDA — 1.5 mg.
Approx. restore — approx. 50 mg. daily

Destroyed By:

alcohol
sugar
clams
fever

Vitamins

    coffee
    stress
    tobacco

Part of the Body Essential For:

    brain
    ears
    eyes
    hair
    heart
    nervous system
    digestive tract
    intestines
    mental ability
    to change glucose into energy or fat
    memory vitamin
    starch-sugar metabolism vitamin
    resistance to noise & pain

Symptoms of Deficiency:

feet & hands numb
lack of hydrochloric acid
low blood pressure
anemia
low metabolic rate
lactic acid build-up
pain, neuritis in legs
water-clogged heart   poor concentration
sciatica   poor circulation
lumbago   nausea
neuralgia   slight paralysis

starved thyroid
pain in knee
delayed ligament
  reflexes

beri-beri
fatigue
constipation

Nutrients Which Augment:
>Vitamin B2
>Folic Acid
>B-Complex
>Niacin
>Vitamins C, E
>Manganese
>Sulphur

Foods & Sources:
>bladderwrack
>dulse
>kelp
>fenugreek
>grape leaves
>red raspberries
>okra
>wheat germ
>asparagus
>whole wheat
>oatmeal
>brown rice
>rice polishings
>potatoes
>beans

peas — 1 c = 4.5 mg
sunflower seeds — 1 c = 2.84 mg
yeast — 1 T = 1.25 mg
green leafy vegetables

Useful For:

alcoholism
congestive heart failure
anemia
nausea
mental illness
rapid heart
stress

Nervous tissue depends on Vitamin B1 for growth and development. Too much white flour and white rice can be the cause of a Thiamin deficiency. Every 100 grams of brown rice contains 2.93 mg. White rice for the same amount has only .60 mg.

Cooking vegetables in too much water, then throwing away the water causes a loss of Thiamin.

More is needed in older ages. Alcoholics can become very deficient. Brain damage can occur from a deficiency.

VITAMIN B2 (Riboflavin) (water soluble)

Daily dose — RDA — 1.7 mg.
Approx. restore — 2-10 mg.

Destroyed By:

alcohol
sugar
clams
fever
coffee
stress
tobacco

light
ultraviolet rays
cooking
antibiotics
oral contraceptives

Parts of the Body Essential For:

blood
nerves
bring oxygen to eyes
milk sugar or lactose increases
need for B2 unless fat is adequate in diet
cell respiration
metabolism of fats, carbohydrates and
   protein

Symptoms of Deficiency:

cracks at corner of mouth
whistle lines
loss of upper lip
swollen eyelids
sensitive to light
eyelids itch & burn
watery eyes

Vitamins

poor night vision
bloodshot eyes
cataracts, glaucoma
blood vessels close to skin, red as in alcoholics, etc.
bed sores
liver impairment
anemia
nervousness
poor digestion

Nutrients Which Augment:

B Complex
B6
Niacin
Phosphorus
Vitamin C

Foods & Sources:

bladderwrack
dulse
fenugreek
kelp
saffron
wild rose hips
veal
asparagus
beets
brussel sprouts

lettuce
barley
bananas
figs
strawberries
watermelon
whole grains
peas
lima beans
sunflower seeds

carrots
cauliflower

brewers yeast
green leafy vegetables

Useful For:

    acne
    cataracts
    mouth sores
    itchy eyes
    digestion

Riboflavin is essential for protein metabolism. A lack of B 2 is one of the causes of birth defects such as skeletal abnormalities, abnormal development of bones such as cleft palate and jaw. It also causes pregnancy deficiencies.

The fetal damage potential is greater when certain drugs are taken. Even when the mother apparently has enough for herself, deficiency with the fetus can cause deformities.

VITAMIN B6 (pyridoxin) (water soluble)

    Daily dose — RDA — 1.8 mg.
    Approx. restore — 4.50 mg.

Destroyed by:

birth control pills
coffee
alcohol
radiation
tobacco

freezing
storage
canning
processing grain
    cooking

Vitamins

Parts of the Body Essential For:

    essential to use fatty acids, linoleic acids & amino acids from protein
    assists in hormonal metabolism of thyrroid, pancreas & adrenal glands
    antibody formation
    digestion
    fat & protein utilization
    maintains sodium & potassium balance
    nerves
    necessary for syntheses of DNA & RNA

Symptoms of Deficiency:

exzema in babies
acne, psoriasis
skin dermatitis, wrinkles
fainting easily
sore mouth
muscle cramps
bed wetting
bladder retention
tooth decay
sinus problem
water retention
toxemia in pregnancy
hemorrhoids
ear noise
nausea in pregnancy — up to 250 mg.

sea sickness, motions sickness- up to 250 mg.
irradiation sickness - to 250 mg.
rheumatism
colitis

B6 levels decline with age

Nutrients Which Augment:

B complex
B1
B2
Pantothenic acid
Vitamin C
Magnesium
Potassium
Sodium

Foods & Sources:

chicken
veal
asparagus
beets
brussel sprouts
carrots
cauliflower
lettuce
barley
bananas
figs

chicken
whole grains
walnuts
filberts
peanuts
sunflower seeds
wheat germ
strawberries
watermelon

Useful For:

arteriosclerosis
baldness
mental retardation
muscular disorders
nervousness

>   stress
>   overweight
>   sensitivity to light or sun
>   skin problems

More Vitamin B6 is needed during pregnancy and old age. Leg cramps during pregnancy are thought to be a lack in calcium and magnesium. Often it is the lack of B6.

Often puffiness and sore breasts before menstruation are lack of B6.

VITAMIN B12 (Cyanocobalamin-Cobalt) (water soluble)

>   Daily dose — RDA — 3 mcg.
>   Approx. restore — 5-50 mcg.

Destroyed by:

>   **alcohol**
>   **coffee**
>   **laxatives**
>   **tobacco**

Parts of the Body essential For:

>   glands
>   phenobarbitol & dilantin & heat destroy folic acid. Folid acid is necessary to use B12. This is a good reason for using

raw cold-pressed oils & raw fruits and
nuts
essential in use of meat protein
essential to gland restoration
where meat is used
blood   nerves

Symptoms of Deficiency:

Inability to produce hydrochloric acid
sore mouth, swollen tongue
bright red, painful tongue
spinal cord degeneration
menstrual disturbances
back stiffness & pain
eyelids painful & burning
vaginal itching
loss of distance vision
red scaley spots between nose & lips
pale
white lips

abdominal difficulties	heart failure
nausea	vomiting
gas	pain
constipation	poor appetite
diarrhea	ringing ears
fatigue	spots before eyes
sleepy	enlarged liver &
irritability	spleen

Nutrients Which Augment

    B Complex
    B6
    Choline
    Inositol
    Vitamin C
    Potassium
    Sodium

Foods & Sources:

    cheese
    cottage cheese
    liver — ¼ lb = 90 mcg
    eggs
    milk
    sea vegetation

Useful For:

    alcoholism
    allergies
    arthritis
    bronchial asthma
    irregular menstrual periods
    stress
    bursitis
    epilepsy

BIOTIN (Vitamin H) (water soluble - part of B-Complex)

Daily dose — RDA — 150-300 mcg.
Approx. restore — 300-500 mcg.

Destroyed by:

alcohol
coffee
raw egg white

Parts of the Body Essential For:

hair
cell growth
cell longevity
vitamin B utilization

Symptoms of Deficiency:

dry skin
gray skin
muscular pain
poor appetite
eczema
dermatitis
leg cramps
mental depression
heart pain
hands & feet tingle
pallor

Vitamins

Nutrients Which Augment:
>B Complex
>B12
>Folic Acid
>Vitamin C
>Sulphur

Foods & Sources:
>soy beans, 1 c = 120 mcg
>lentils, 1 c = 25 mcg
>bean sprouts, 1 c = 200 mcg
>yeast
>cheese
>brown rice
>rolled oats
>milk
>nuts

Useful For:
>baldness
>dermatitis
>exzema
>leg cramps

CHOLINE (part of B-Complex - water soluble)
>Daily dose — RDA — None
>Approx. restore — 1,000-10,000 mcg

Destroyed by:
>sugar (excessive)
>coffee
>alcohol

Parts of the Body Essential For:
>keeps arteries clear
>lecithin formation
>liver, gall bladder regulation
>metabolism (fats & cholesterol)
>nerve transmission
>thymus

Symptoms of Deficiency:

>without choline, cholesterol reaches high levels because it takes choline to produce lecithin. Damage to kidneys result from lack of choline when protein diet is used.

Nutrients Which Augment:
>Vitamins A, B Complex B12
>Folic Acid
>Linoleic acid
>Inositol
>Lecithin

Foods & Sources:
    peanuts, ½ c = 190 mcg
    soy oil
    wheat germ oil

Useful For:
    alcoholism
    arteriosclerosis
    baldness
    high cholesterol
    constipation
    dizziness
    ear noise
    hardening of the arteries
    heart trouble
    headaches
    high blood pressure
    hypoglycemia
    insomnia

Mother's milk has a choline-lecithin balance for humans, which cows milk does not. Therefore, nursing mothers give their children an immune ability which a bottle fed baby does not have.

Choline has an effect on the thymus glands also, which in turn has something to do with growth and immune response in a child.

FOLIC ACID (Part of B-Complex - water soluble)

Daily dose — RDA — 400 mcg
Approx. restore — 1,000 - 10,000 mcg

Destroyed by:

birth control pills
alcohol
coffee
stress
tobacco
cooking, dissolves in water
air
light

Parts of the Body Essential For:

synthesis of DNA & other nucleic acids
appetite
body growth & reproduction
hydrochloric acid production
protein metabolism, red blood cell
    formation
growth of cells

Symptoms of Deficiency:

anemia
digestive disturbances
graying hair
growth problems

Vitamins

    pregnancy cap
    skin dryness
    joints dry
    diarrhea
    afterbirth hemorrhage
    mental illness

Nutrients Which Augment:

    B Complex
    B12
    Biotin
    Pantothenic acid
    Vitamin C

Foods & Sources:

    dates, 1 med = 2500 mcg
    spinach, 1 c = 448 mcg
    wheat bran
    beet greens
    kale
    endive
    turnips
    potatoes
    broccoli
    orange juice
    swiss chard
    black-eyed peas
    lima beans
    asparagus

Useful For:
>alcoholism
anemia
arteriosclerosis
baldness
diarrhea
fatigue
mental illness
stomach ulcers
stress
healing
use of vitamin B12
pregnancy

>Elderly people suffer from deficiency.

INOSITOL (Part of B-complex - water soluble)
>Daily dose — RDA — none
Approx. restore — 100-1000 mg.

Destroyed by:
>alcohol
coffee

Parts of the Body Essential For:
>lecithin formation
metabolism of fats
hair growth

reduces cholesterol
retards artery hardening
has an inhibiting factor in cancer
has been used for nerve damage in MS, but must be used in conjunction with Vitamin E
when used with choline, breaks up fat

Symptoms of Deficiency:

high cholesterol
exzema
hair loss
eye problems

Nutrients Which Augment:

B Complex
B12
Choline
Linoleic acid
Vitamin E

Foods & Sources:

wheat germ
oranges, 1 med = 400 mg
grapefruit, 1 med = 500 mg
peanuts, 1 c = 400 mg
brown rice
citrus fruit
brewers yeast
molasses

Useful For:
>arteriosclerosis
baldness
high cholesterol
heart disease
overweight

NIACIN (Vitamin B3, Part of B-Complex - water soluble)
>Daily Dose — RDA — 13-18 mg
Approx. restore — 50 - 5,000 mg

Destroyed by:
>alcohol
antibiotics
coffee
corn sugar
excessive starch
cooking

Parts of the Body Essential For:
>circulation
reduces cholesterol
growth
hydrochloric acid production
metabolism of proteins, cabohydrates, & starches
sex hormone production

Vitamins

Symptoms of Deficiency:

appetite loss
canker sores
depression
fatigue
halitosis
headaches
indigestion
insomnia
muscle weakness
nausea
skin eruptions
nervous problems
fear
neuralgia
diarrhea
coated tongue
impaired memory
schizophrenia

tongue deep red with fissures. (fissures will turn black if great deficiency. Becomes pellagra or Black Tongue (plague) rash on neck & forearms

Nutrients Which Augment:

B Complex
Vitamins B1, B2, C
Phosphorus

Foods & Sources:

peanuts, 1c = 40 mg
rhubarb, cooked, 80 mg
whole wheat
sunflower seeds, 1c = **7.8 mg**

brewers yeast, 1T = 3 mg
peas, 1 c = 3.7 mg

Useful For:
- senility
- cataracts
- acne
- baldness
- halitosis
- high blood pressure
- leg cramps
- migraine headache
- tooth decay

Niacin dilates blood vessels and causes hot flash. It is used to increase circulation to the brain in senility, schizophrena and ear and eye problems.

It is also useful for alcoholics and reduces cholesterol levels. It has been used to treat pellagra, black tongue and fissures of the tongue. Women are more subject to this than men.

PANTHOTHENIC ACID (part of B-complex — anti-stress vitamin — water soluble)

Daily Dose — RDA .05-10 mg
Approx. restore — 20-100 mg.

Vitamins

Destroyed by:
- coffee
- alcohol
- methyl bromide

Parts of the Body Essential For:
- anti-body formations
- carbohydrate, fat & protein conversion to energy
- vitamin utilization
- lymph glands
- adrenals
- tonsils

Symptoms of Deficiency:
- arthritis
- hypoglycemia
- exhaustion
- blackouts
- headache
- nervousness
- dizziness
- digestive problems
- depression
- colitis
- cataracts
- low blood pressure
- swollen glands
- glaucoma

gastritis
ulcers
gout
muscle cramps
stretch marks
grinding teeth

Nutrients Which Augment:

B complex
Vitamins B6, B12, C
Biotin
Folic Acid
PABA

Foods & Sources:

whole wheat & bran
mushrooms, 1 c = 25 mg
elderberries, 1 c = 82 mg.
orange juice, 1 c = 45 mg
sesame seeds
brewers yeast
sunflower seeds
soy beans
peas
peanuts

Useful For:

allergies
arthritis

baldness
cystitis
digestive disorders
stress
tooth decay
hypoglycemia
healing:
    cold sores
    sinus
    asthma
    respiratory flu
    colds
relief of gas
used as a fumigator

PABA (Para-Amino-benzoic-acid — part of B complex - water soluble)

Daily Dose — RDA — none
Approx. restore — 10-100 mg

Destroyed by:

alcohol
coffee
sulfa drug

Parts of the Body Essential For:

blood cell formation
gray hair restoration
headaches
irritability

Symptoms of Deficiency:

    digestive disturbances
    graying hair
    irritability
    fatigue
    depression

Nutrients Which Augment:

    B complex
    Folic acid
    Vitamin C
    Pantothenic acid

Foods & Sources:

    blackstrap molasses
    brewers yeast
    wheat germ

    PABA can only be synthesized by intestinal bacteria & stimulates intestinal bacteria to produce folic acid. It is also involved somehow in the utilization of pantothenic acid

Useful For:

    baldness
    gray hair
    overactive thyroid
    parasitic disease
    rheumatic fever

Vitamins

> stress
> infertility
> burns
> dry skin
> sunburn
> wrinkles
> skin spots
> Rocky Mtn. Spotted fever, approx. 1,000 mg daily
> hair color restored — approx 200 mg after each meal
> PABA performs the same thing in the body that sulfa drug does, killing bacteria, without the side effects of sulfa: extreme fatigue, anemia, exzema

PANGAMIC ACID (Part of B complex — B15 — not sold in US at present)

> Daily Dose — RDA — none
> Approx. restore — not known

Destroyed by:

> alcohol
> coffee

Parts of the Body Essential For:

> cell oxidation and respiration
> metabolism of proteins, fats & starches
> glandular & nervous system stimulation

Symptoms of Deficiency:
>heart problems
>nervousness
>gland malfunction

Nutrients Which Augment:
>B Complex
>Vitamins C, E

Foods & Sources
>Brewer's yeast
>brown rice
>seeds — sunflower, pumpkin, sesame
>almonds

Useful For:
>alcoholism
>asthma
>arteriosclerosis
>high cholesterol
>emphysema
>heart disease
>headache
>insomnia
>poor circulation
>premature aging
>rheumatism
>shortness of breath

VITAMIN C (ascorbic acid — water soluble)

Daily Dose — RDA — 45 mg
Approx. restore — 250-5000 mg.

Destroyed by:

antibiotics
aspirin
cortisone
stress
tobacco

Parts of the Body Essential For:

bone & teeth formation
digestion
red blood cell formation
prevents hemorrhage
resists shock & colds
cell respiration
breaking down protein
healing
capillary
cartilage & connective tissue

Symptoms of Deficiency:

anemia
bleeding membrane (mouth, red toothbrush)
low blood pressure
nosebleed
loose teeth   disc problems

edema
mononucleosis
wounds will not heal
pigmentation during pregnancy
varicose veins
high cholesterol
hepatitis, liver
rheumatic fever
cataracts
weakness in arteries
glaucoma
cold sores
high blood pressure
adrenal exhaustion
ulcers
arthritis, gout

Nutrients Which Augment:

All vitamins & minerals
Bioflavonoids
calcium
magnesium

Foods & Sources:

Oranges, 1 med = 100 mg
broccoli, 1 c = 135 mg
green peppers, 1 med = 100 mg
grapefruit, 1 med = 100 mg
papaya, raw, 225 mg
strawberries, 1 c = 90 mg
all fruits & most vegetables

Useful For:

sore throat, strep
sinusitis

Vitamins

stress
aspirin poisoning
black widow spider bites
poison oak or ivy
carbon monoxide
radiation poison
broken bones
bruises
burns
poisonous bites
meningitis
encephalitis
virus disease
swollen glands
polio
asthma
respiratory ailments
acute sinus
kidney infection
phlebitis
hay fever
colds
barrier against
bladder cancer

There are many arguments about how man is missing a gene that requires him to get all of his Vitamin C out of his food, since other mammals produce their own Vitamin C plentifully. If science would recognize that man lives better as a fruitarian he could suppose that was why he was made in such a way that would make Vitamin C production unnecessary in his body.

If man took the comparison amounts that other animals produce, he would have to take 20,000 mg. a day. The RDA is only 60 mg. Man was intended to be a fruit eater and if he were, he would probably not need so much Vitamin C to compensate for the stress foods he lives on.

It has been agreed upon by experts that stress destroys Vitamin C and that under stress the adrenal glands output of hormones increases. Collagen or connective tissue requires Vitamin C. Man's body cannot make collagen without Vitamin C. This is why additional Vitamin C is so helpful to the healing process from surgery or injury when tissue repair is essential.

Vitamin C's main function is the reason it detoxifies even the worst poisons — because it dissolves mucus waste and carries it off through the kidneys. Toxic poisons become a part of mucus waste and Vitamin C quickly detoxifies the body from an acid to an alkaline. This is proven in that a cold can be brought on by taking high doses of Vitamin C, breaking up and moving waste from the body. It also has an antibiotic ability to destroy germs.

When Vitamin C is taken in large doses for extended periods, such as a five to ten days, calcium and Vitamin B should be added, as the Vitamin C leaches these elements and causes nervousness and hollow, easily broken bones.

There has been much discussion about Vitamin C. It has been my experience, and the experience of many others that when Vitamin C is issued (1,000 mg. an hour) in acute illnesses such as a cold, etc., it dissolves mucus and usually stops acute disease or inflammation within a day or two. It has been used successfully even with small babies.

Vitamin C has been considered to be harmful to the kidney when taken in high doses. Certainly it is when it is a coal tar product. Taking high doses of coal tar would be very harmful. To determine whether or not your Vitamin C is a coal tar product, you can make this experiment: Place the tablet or powder on a teaspoon with water, hold over the burner of the stove and let it boil. If it boils away to a white powder, it is not a coal tar product. If it boils to a sticky, black gum, it is a coal tar product. Vitamin C has recently been made from wood, and, of course, would be a synthetic. When made from corn and citrus, it is a natural food product. When used in the case of a cold or acute disease, it should be determined just how the Vitamin C you use is made, or you will not get the results. Could this be the reason for the controversy about Vitamin C? I have found where acute disease is present, straight ascorbic acid is best, usually taking it only a day or two, as it dissolves mucus rapidly. Any acute disease brings with it a rapid pulse, as waste is on the move in the blood. High doses of Vitamin C often increases the heartbeat, as with acute disease. The addition of approximately one capsule of cayenne will usually slow down and smooth out the heart. Bioflavinoid Vitamin C is best for a daily dose.

VITAMIN D (Sunshine vitamin — fat soluble)

    Daily Dose — RDA 400 IU
    Approx. restore — 500-1,500 IU

Destroyed by:

    mineral oil

Parts of the Body Essential For:

    calcium & phosphorus metabolism
    bone formation
    heart action
    blood clotting
    skin respiration
    teeth
    growth
    People who do not get out in the sunshine do themselves a great injustice; much mental illness is caused from lack of calcium, and calcium cannot be used without Vitamin D

Vitamins

Symptoms of Deficiency:

burning mouth & throat
insomnia
myopia
nervousness
poor metabolism
soft bones & teeth
fingernails split & deep lines
rickets   bowed legs
ostioporosis   faulty jaw dev
high cholest.   retard. growth
muscle cramps   jt. & back pain
bones break easily
backache
pyorrhea
acne
weakness
enlarged joints

Nutrients Which Augment:

Vitamins A, C, F
Calcium
Phosphorus
Choline

Foods & Sources:

alfalfa
sunlight
cod liver oil
salmon or tuna, ¼ lb = 300 IU

cream
milk (D enriched)
egg yolk
lettuce

Useful For:

alcoholism
arthritis
stress
counteracts drug harm

Vitamin D is stored by the body in the liver during the winter months

VITAMIN E (tocopherol — fat soluble)

Daily Dose — RDA — 12-15 IU
Approx. restore — 50-600 IU

Destroyed by:

estrogen drugs
birth control pills
chlorine
mineral oil
rancid fats & oils
inorganic iron

Parts of the Body Essential For:

aging retardation
anti-clotting factor
lowers cholesterol

Vitamins

  strengths capillary walls
  fertility
  muscle, nerve maintenance
  growth
  nutrition
  essential to use of A, C, D & K
  protects fat tissue from abnormal breakdown as in diabetes
  effective in menopause
  effective in menstrual cramps
  heart
  normal blood pressure
  effective on burns & scars
  healing broken bones
  increases oxygen

Symptoms of Deficiency:

  sterility
  blood clot
  detachment of retina
  heart problems
  anemia
  puffy eyes
  menopause problems
  varicose veins

  Caution: chronic heart (coronary artery disease) approx 800 to 1600 IU daily rheumatic heart approx 90 IU for 3-4 weeks. Then increase to 150 IU. High blood pressure requires careful supervision. Slow results in beginning with eventual great value.

Nutrients Which Augment:

Vitamins A, B1, B, C, F
Manganese
Phosphorus
Inositol
Selenium (trace element)

Foods & Sources:

wheat germ oil, 1 T = 40 IU
safflower oil, 1 T = 20 IU
oats   peanuts
rice   broccoli
green leafy vegetables
nettle leaves, 1 lb = 98.2

Useful For:

detached retina   congenital heart
premature babies   acne
anemia   cancer cell growth
hernia   skin cancer
muscle weakness   hemophilia
crossed eyes   sinus
miscarriage   arthritis
burns & scars   colitis
varicose veins   arteriosclerosis
frostbite   gallstones
pain   hepatitis

clots
heart attack
thyroid gland
stomach ulcers
elimination of poison

hot flashes
drug abuse
maintaining youth
energy & endurance

VITAMIN F (unsaturated fatty acid — fat soluble)

Daily Dose — RDA — none
Approx. restore — 10% total calorie intake

Destroyed by:

radiation
X-ray

Parts of the Body Essential For:

prevents hardening of arteries
normalizes blood pressure
gland activity

Symptoms of Deficiency:

acne
brittle nails
eczema
gall stones
brittle hair
underweight
varicose veins

Nutrients Which Augment:
>Vitamins A, C, D. E
>Phosphorus

Foods & Sources:
>vegetable oils
>wheat germ
>sunflower seeds

Useful For:
>allergies
>baldness
>bronchial asthma
>eczema
>gallbladder problems
>leg ulcers
>psoriasis
>overweight
>rheumatoid arthritis

VITAMIN K (menadione — fat soluble)
>Daily Dose — RDA — none
>Approx. restore — 300-500 mcg

Destroyed by:
>drugs
>aspirin
>antibiotics

Vitamins

>   mineral oils
>   radiation
>   rancid fats
>   x-rays

Parts of the Body Essential For:

>   clotting of blood

Symptoms of Deficiency:

>   hemophilia
>   hemorrhages easily
>   nosebleeds
>   diarrhea

Nutrients Which Augment:

>   are not known

Foods & Sources:

>   green leafy vegetables
>   safflower oil
>   blackstrap molasses
>   alfalfa
>   chestnuts
>   shepherds purse
>   cabbage
>   cauliflower
>   plantain
>   spinach
>   potatoes
>   soy beans

tomatoes
potatoes
peas
carrots

Useful For:
bruising
eye hemorrhage
gallstones
menstrual problems
preparing for childbirth
hemorrhage

Vitamin K is synthesized or manufactured by intestinal bacteria. It is, therefore, necessary to maintain natural flora in the bowel — antibiotics destroy this flora.

Vitamin K is used when patient has been on long term antibiotics of intravenous feeding for more than seven days.

VITAMIN P (bioflavonoids)
Daily Dose — RDA — none
Approx. restore — 500-3,000 mg

Destroyed by:
Same as Vitamin C

Parts of the Body Essential For:
- blood vessel walls
- connective tissue
- skin
- prevention of flu & colds
- strengthens capillaries
- minimizes bruising

Symptoms of Deficiency:
- same as Vitamin C
- uterine bleeding
- irregular menstrual flow where no other cause is known
- varicose veins

Nutrients Which Augment:
- Vitamin C

Foods & Sources:
- skins & pulp of fruits
- buckwheat
- paprika
- rue
- apricots
- cantaloupe
- broccoli
- papaya
- cherries
- tomatoes

green peppers

Useful For:

- asthma
- bleeding gums
- colds
- eczema
- dizziness
- high blood pressure
- miscarriage
- rheumatic fever
- rheumatism
- ulcers
- hemorrhoids
- veins
- capillaries
- RH babies to strengthen veins & arteries for blood change

The rest of the C complex necessary on a daily intake of minimum dose — used as a preventative. Straight Vitamin C (abscorbic acid) in high doses work faster for acute disease, but the full C complex should be used on a regular basis.

SECTION II

MINERALS

CALCIUM
    Daily Dose — RDA — 800-1400 mg
    Approx. restore — 1,000-2,000 mg

Destroyed by:
- lack of exercise
- stress

Parts of the Body Essential For:
- bone & tooth formation
- blood clotting
- heart rhythm
- nerve tranquilizing
- nerve transmission
- muscle growth
- lactation & pregnancy
- oxygen to brain
- muscle contraction

Symptoms of Deficiency:

menstrual cramps   cyst formations

tooth decay
night sweats
leg cramps
mental depression
irritability
brooding, complaining
tooth grinding
nervousness

sores do not heal
lack of courage
soft bones
deterioration of
   spine
sleeplessness
muscle cramps
tooth decay

Nutrients Which Augment:

    Vitamins A, C, D, F
    Iron
    Magnesium
    Manganese
    Phosphorus

Foods & Sources:

(abundance)
poultry
cottage cheese
swiss cheese
artichokes
lima beans
beets, leaves & root
broccoli
brussel sprouts
carrots
celery

okra
rutabaga
sauerkraut
squash
whole wheat bread
hominy

figs
peaches
coconut
filberts

Minerals

(some)
- beef
- lamb
- liver
- veal
- buttermilk
- cream
- eggs
- parsley
- parsnips
- peas
- potatoes
- rhubarb
- tomatoes
- turnips, tops & root
- watercress
- rye bread
- corn
- rice
- rye
- walnuts
- asparagus
- cauliflower
- endive
- sesame
- tahini
- carob
- beans
- wheat
- apples
- avocados
- bananas
- blueberries
- dates
- olives
- oranges
- raisins
- raspberries
- hickory nuts
- peanuts

Useful For:

- arthritis
- aging symptoms
- bachache
- foot & leg cramps
- insomnia
- menstrual cramps
- pain
- dental pain
- heart
- skin
- kidney
- brain
- muscles
- liver

menopause   spleen
overweight   bones
rheumatism   hair
delivery   teeth
bites
broken bones

CHROMIUM

    Daily Dose — RDA — none
    Approx. restore — 100-300 mcg

Destroyed by:

    refining process

Parts of the Body Essential For:

    normal blood sugar levels
    glucose metabolism

Symptoms of Deficiency:

    arteriosclerosis
    glucose intolerance in diabetes
    growth inhibited
    high cholesterol
    hyperglycemia
    hypoglycemia

Nutrients Which Augment:

    none known

Minerals

Foods & Sources:
> sea vegetation
> corn oil
> brewers yeast
> grains
> fresh fruits & vegetables

Useful For:
> diabetes
> hypoglycemia
> improvement of insulin balance

COBALT
> Daily Dose — RDA — 100 mcg
> Approx. restore — 100-300 mcg

Destroyed by:
> Not known

Parts of the Body Essential For:
> Not known

Symptoms of Deficiency:
> pernicious anemia
> slow growth
> anemia
> nervous disorder

Nutrients Which Augment:
>Vitamin B12
>Folic acid

Foods & Sources:
>cheese
>fish
>eggs
>wheat germ
>yeast
>comfrey leaves

Useful For:
>pregnancy
>lactation

COPPER (trace mineral)
>Daily Dose — RDA — 2 mg
>Approx. restore — 2-4 mg

Destroyed by:
>zinc — high intake

Parts of the Body Essential For:
>bone formation
>hair & skin color
>healing processes
>hemoglobin & blood cell formation

Minerals

Symptoms of Deficiency:
    general weakness
    impaired respiration
    skin sores
    grey hair

Nutrients Which Augment:
    Cobalt
    Vitamin C
    Iron
    Zinc

Foods & Sources:
    brazil nuts, 4 mg
    soybeans, 1c = 2 mg
    almonds
    prunes
    lima beans
    broccoli
    wheat bran
    navy beans
    kidney beans
    apricots
    avocados
    corn
    figs
    currants
    filberts
    widespread through all foods

Useful For:
> anemia
> baldness

> Copper accumulates in the blood when there is no iron, eventually causing Wilson's Disease

IODINE

> Daily Dose — RDA — 100-130 mcg
> Approx. restore — 100-1000 mcg

Destroyed by:
> Vitamin C

Parts of the Body Essential For:
> hair
> skin
> teeth
> nails
> speech
> mentality

Symptoms of Deficiency:
> cold hands & feet
> dry hair
> irritability
> nervousness

Minerals

obesity
difficult birth
hardening of arteries
goiter

Nutrients Which Augment:

Sodium

Foods & Sources:

sea vegetation
seafood
turnips, root
peppers
kelp
dulse-deep sea lettuce
carrots
broccoli
raw goat milk
asparagus
potatoes
beans
chard
turnip greens
spinach

Useful For:

arteriosclerosis
hair problem
goiter
hyperthyroidism

childbirth
lactation
infection
inflamation

losses occur during summer - perspiration

IRON

Daily Dose — RDA — 10-18 mg.
Approx. restore — 15-50 mg.

Destroyed by:

pain drugs
coffee
excess phosphorus
tea
zinc - excessive

Parts of the Body Essential For:

disease resistance
muscles
blood
oxygen
bone marrow

Symptoms of Deficiency:

cry involuntarily
lack oxygen

Minerals

anemia
blood lacks color
decreased energy
weakness
dizziness
short breath
pounding heart
palpitations
fatigue
brittle fingernails with
 longitudinal ridging, colorlessness
lacking vitality
forgetfulness
pain in heels
dull hearing
sleepless at night
arthritis

Nutrients Which Augment:

Vitamin B6
B12
Folic acid
Copper
Cobalt
Phosphorus
Calcium
Vitamin C

Foods & Sources:

blackstrap molasses

pumpkin
green leafy veg.
dried fruits
alfalfa
sea vegetation
beans
seeds
wheat germ
small amt in all foods

Useful For:

aids blood cells
development of tissue respiration
oxygen transportation
alcoholism
anemia
colitis
menstrual period
pregnancy
lactation
Iron function

recycles except during menstruation or hemorrhage
not absorbed without hydrocholin, or when taking alkalizing preparations.
destroys Vitamin E — take 8 hrs. apart

MAGNESIUM

Daily Dose — RDA — 300-350 mg
Approx. restore — 300-1000 mg

Destroyed by:

cortisone
antibiotics
milk
cooked nuts
white bread
x-ray

Parts of the Body Essential For:

preserving mineral balance
utilization of calcium
acid alkaline balance
blood sugar balance
metabolism of Vitamin C

Symptoms of Deficiency:

confusion
disorientation
anger
nervousness
rapid pulse
tremors
bed wetting
fear
gas
insomnia
hyperactivity
convulsions
colitis
diarrhea
kidney stones
muscle ache & pain
mental disorders
anxiety

palpitations of heart   prostate problems
yellowish white in eyes
muscle spasms, twitching
sensitive to noise   suicidal tendency
edema   senility

Nutrients Which Augment:

    Vitamin B6, C, D
    Calcium
    Phosphorus

Foods & Sources:

peanuts, 1 c = 420 mg

lettuce leaf	onions
tomatoes	peas
watercress	potatoes
corn	spinach
leeks	sauerkraut
parsnips	turnips
alfalfa	barley
lentils	rye
mushrooms	wheat

mustard greens
small amt. in most foods

    alcoholism
    high cholesterol
    depression
    heart condition

Minerals

       kidney stones
       prostate troubles
       stomach acidity
       tooth decay
       overweight
       blood vessels
       healthy nervous system
       calcium utilization
       heart
       glands
       spinal fluid
       brain

When the pituitary is not getting necessary magnesium, it fails in its regulatory function for the adrenals, allowing them to over produce, resulting in anxiety and seeming nervousness.

When the adrenals become exhausted from overproduction of adrenal hormones, low blood sugar and inability to cope with stress are the result.

Milk depletes magnesium because the synthetic Vitamin D found in milk binds magnesium. Children who have epilepsy or tendency to convulsions only increase the risk by drinking milk.

Magnesium is necessary in high altitudes to lessen the effort of the heart which must work harder because the small vessels of the lungs tend to constrict in high altitudes. Magnesium makes a change in the process of such constriction.

Processed foods could be the cause of exhausted people with so many nervous afflictions and with distorted thinking, because magnesium is destroyed in the processing of foods.

MANGANESE
    Daily Dose — RDA — none
    Approx. restore — 1.5 mg.

Destroyed by:
    Choline
    Calcium (excessive)
    Phosphorus (excessive)
    Biotin

Parts of the Body Essential For:
    activation of enzymes
    reproduction & growth
    hormone production
    tissue repair
    Vitamins B1 & E utilization
    important in growth, pregnancy & lactation

brain
muscles
nerves

Symptoms of Deficiency:
multiple sclerosis
muscle coordination failure
dizziness
ear noise
loss of hearing

Nutrients Which Augment:
None

Foods & Sources:
pineapple
bananas
celery
peas, dried
barley
turnips
almonds
brazil nuts
swiss cheese
corn
beans
beet root
kale
raspberries

nuts
bran
blueberries

Useful For:
allergies
asthma
diabetes
fatigue
multiple sclerosis
growth
reproduction
bones
teeth
central nervous system

PHOSPHORUS
Daily Dose — RDA — 800 mg
Approx. restore — 800-1,000 mg

Destroyed by:
antacids
aluminum
iron
magnesium (excessive)
white sugar (excessive)

Parts of the Body Essential For:
bone & teeth formation

cell growth & repair
energy
heart muscles contraction
kidney function
metabolism of calcium & sugar
nerve & muscle activity
vitamin utilization, esp. B
nursing mothers
development of cells
metabolism of fats
necessary for mental power

Symptoms of Deficiency:

afraid of tomorrow
dislike sex, work
fearful
general weakness
loss of muscle tone
numbness of limbs
prone to arthritis
paralysis
appetite loss
fatigue
irregular breathing
overweight or weight loss
tooth decay
poor growth of hair
poor growth of fingernails

Nutrients Which Augment:
> Vitamins A, D, F
> Calcium
> Iron
> Manganese

Foods & Sources:
> milk
> yogurt, 1 c = 250 mg.
> eggs, 1 med = 110 mg.

Useful For:
> arthritis
> stress
> tooth & gum disorders
> retarded growth in children

Phosphorus is not properly absorbed without sufficient hydrochloric acid in the stomach. With adrenal insufficiency or low blood sugar, phosphorus may not be used. (see "Is Any Sick Among You" for information on hormone herbs.)

POTASSIUM
> Daily Dose — RDA — None
> Approx. restore — 3,000-10,000 mg.

Minerals

Destroyed by:
- too much sodium
- alcohol
- coffee
- cortisone
- too many laxitives
- excessive sugar
- stress
- salt
- diuretics
- drug hormones

Parts of the Body Essential For:
- alkalinity of body fluids
- normal heartbeat
- body growth
- muscle contraction
- nerve tranquilization
- proper functions of digestion

Symptoms of Deficiency:
- hypoglycemia
- acne
- continuous thirst
- dry skin
- constipation
- general weakness
- insomnia
- muscle damage

nervousness
slow, irregular heartbeat
weak reflexes
water retention
weak ligaments
listlessness
soft, flabby muscles
swollen testicles or ovaries

Nutrients Which Augment:

Vitamin B6
Sodium

Foods & Sources:

apricots, dried, 1 c = 1450 mg
bananas, 1 med = 500 mg
sunflowerseeds, 1 c = 900 mg.
(abundant)

celery	beef
gooseberries	brazil nuts
cucumbers	eggs
kale	(some)
lettuce	cream
cooked onions	cheese
cooked onions	molasses
sweet potatoes	broccoli
pumpkin	carrots
radishes	cabbage
rutabaga	cauliflower
squash	chard

Minerals

tomatoes
watercress
oatmeal
rice
apricots
blueberries
cherries
cranberries
buttermilk
dates
figs
peaches
prunes
watermelon
hickory nuts
barley
peanuts
apples
salmon
pineapples
strawberries

eggplant
endive
lentils
leeks
mushroom
mustard greens
onions
parsley
haddock
parsnips
peas
walnuts
sauerkraut
spinach
turnips, tops & roots
chestnuts
rye
avocados
corn
limes
herring   lamb

Useful For

acne
allergies
diabetes

alcoholism
colic
high blood pressure

Leakage of potassium from cells or loss of potassium could be the cause of muscular distophy, as potassium is necessary for muscle strength.

Losses occur by:
>spilling off in urine
>too much sodium intake
>dieuretics (water pills)
>ATCH
>cortisone
>aspirin
>drugs
>alcohol
>drinking too much water
>vomiting
>diarrhea
>stress

Excessive sugar causes stress, spilling off potassium. This could be more the cause of heart attack than too many fatty acids. Sugar decreases cell potassium, rendering heart and all muscles weak and flabby.

Another reason for heart weakness is the use of too much salt. If the intake is no more than 1 tsp. daily, at least 5,000 mg of potassium is required. We Americans consume at least 1 to 5 tsp. of salt daily and do not eat enough fruits and vegetables to make up for the potassium deficiency.

Potassium has been noticeably lacking in leukemia and polio patients. Diabetics lose potassium when high sugar is ingested, causing a potassium deficiency.

SILICON

Daily Dose — RDA — unknown
Approx. restore —

Destroyed by:
Not known

Parts of the Body Essential For:
natural alkalizer
regulate cell tissue

Symptoms of Deficiency:
itchy ears
sties on eyes
ear discharge
ulceration of tongue
sensitive teeth
boils
nervous exhaustion
listlessness
no ambition for brain work

Foods & Sources:
apricots
cherries
endive
cauliflower
asparagus

lima beans
parsley
pumpkin
horseradish
lettuce
oranges
olives
almonds
coconut
current
beets
persimmons
horsetail

Useful For:

drug addiction

SODIUM

Daily Dose — RDA — 3000-7000 mg.
Approx. restore — 3000-10,000 mg.

Destroyed by:

chlorine
lack of potassium

Parts of the Body Essential For:

normal cellular fluid
muscle contraction

Minerals

Symptoms of Deficiency:

appetite loss
muscle shrinkage
intestinal gas
vomiting
weight loss
low blood pressure
heat stroke when in sun too long
heat stroke symptoms: nausea, dizziness, exhaustion, vomiting, cramp of leg, back or abdominal muscles being used at the time
hair falling out
loss of sense of smell
indigestion
early morning exhaustion

Nutrients Which Augment:

Vitamin D
Potassium

Foods & Sources:

(abundant)
grapes
olives
pears
brazil nuts
peanuts
walnuts
herring
prunes
strawberries
watermelon
chestnuts
cocoanut
swiss cheese
asparagus
beans

limberger cheese
raw goat milk
molasses
alfalfa
kale
leeks
rutabaga
sauerkraut
squash
turnips
barley
eggs
pomegranate (some)
blueberries
cherries
cranberries
dates
gooseberries
lemons
limes
pineapple

celery
beets
dill
carrots
cauliflower
chard
endive
lettuce
okra
parsley
peas
potatoes
rhubarb
tomatoes
watercress
corn
rice
wheat
apples
avocado
bananas
egg yolk

Useful For:
dehydration
fever
heat stroke
natural alkalizer
regulating cell tissues
There is a big difference in sodium as it occurs naturally in food, than sodium chloride or salt.

SULPHUR

Daily Dose — RDA — none
Approx. restore — trace

Destroyed by:
not known

Parts of the Body Essential For:
body tissue formation
toning blood
improving looks
stimulating liver secretions
called beautifying mineral

Symptoms of Deficiency:
toxic condition
disc trouble
hair dull
joint troubles
joyless appearance
difficulty talking or singing
menstruation delayed
menstruation irregular
moodiness
sores do not heal
voicebox gives out easily

Nutrients Which Augment:
Vitamin B1

B Complex
Biotin
Pantothenic acide

Sulfur of the type not occuring naturally in food is poison to the body. This type is used to sulfur fruits to preserve color.

Foods & Sources:

(abundant)
nuts
wheat germ
poultry
veal
raw goat milk
asparagus
carrots
cauliflower
endive
lettuce
parsnips
potatoes
peaches
whole wheat
corn
rice
bananas
dates
figs
olives

lentils
mushrooms
mustard greens
cooked onions
parsley
peas
peppers
sweet potatoes
raisins
pumpkin
radishes
rhubarb
rutabaga
sauerkraut
tomatoes
turnips
watercress
barley
wheat germ
apricots
blueberries

Minerals

oranges
watermelon
hickory nuts
peanuts
(some)
butter
cheese
molasses
soybeans
lima beans
beets
broccoli
celery
chard
eggplant

blackberries
cantaloupe
cherries
cranberries
gooseberries
grapefruit
grapes
lemons
limes
raspberries
coconut
filberts
pecans
walnuts

Useful For:

arthritis
external skin disorders
muscles
brain
skin
bones

ZINC

Daily Dose — RDA — 15 mg.
Approx. restore — 20-100 mg.

Destroyed by:

    alcohol
    calcium (high intake)
    lack of phosphorus

Parts of the Body Essential For:

    burns & wound healing
    carbohydrate digestion
    prostate gland function
    reproductive organ growth
      & development
    sex organ growth & development
    Vitamin B1, phosphorus & protein
      metabolism

Symptoms of Deficiency:

    delayed sexual maturity
    fatigue
    loss of taste
    poor appetite
    slow healing of wounds
    retarded growth
    sterility

Nutrients Which Augment:

    Vitamin A
    Calcium
    Copper

Phosphorus

Foods & Sources:

    brewers yeast
    soybeans
    spinach
    sunflower seeds
    mushrooms
    green leafy veg.
    bran
    wheat germ
    onions
    maple syrup

Useful For:

    alcoholism
    arteriosclerosis
    cirrhosis
    diabetes
    wounds
    high cholesterol
    infertility

DNA molecules are the principles of all life forms on earth. When anything is alive it has DNA molecules. This is the characteristic which makes it possible to form new cells and grow.

DNA give instruction and RNA or ribonucleic acid, does the work, or carries out the genetic plan. Zinc is necessary for DNA to function properly.

SECTION III
Vitamin & Mineral Deficiences & Diseases

ACNE
Vitamin A
Niacin
Potassium
Sulphur
Vitamin B2
Vitamin E

ALCOHOLISM
Pangamic acid
Folic acid
B Complex
Potassium
Zinc
Choline

ALLERGIES
Pantothenic acid
B Complex
Potassium
Manganese
Vitamin F

ANEMIA
Folic acid
B Complex
Vitamin B1
Iron
Copper
Vitamin E

APPETITE LOSS
Zinc
Biotin

ARTERIOSCLEROSIS
Vitamin A
Choline

ARTHRITIS
Pantothenic acid
B Complex
Phosphorus
Sulphur
Calcium
Vitamin F
Vitamin E

ASPIRIN POISONING
Vitamin C

ATHEROSCLEROSIS
Iodine
Pangemic acid
Inositol
Folic acid
Zinc
Vitamin B6
Choline
Vitamin F
Biotin

BALDNESS
Paba
Pantothenic acid
Niacin
Inositol
Folic acid
B Complex

Vitamin B6
Biotin
Copper
Vitamin F

BARBITURATE OVERDOSE
B Complex

BLACK WIDOW SPIDER BITES
Vitamin C

BLEEDING GUMS
Vitamin P
Vitamin C

BLOOD CLOTS
Vitamin E

BROKEN BONES
Vitamin E
Calcium
Vitamin C

BRUISES
Vitamin C
Vitamin K

BURNS
Vitamin C
Zinc
Paba
Vitamin E

CARBON MONOXIDE POISONING
Vitamin C

CATARACTS
Niacin
Vitamin B2

CIRRHOSIS
Zinc

COLD HANDS & FEET
Iodine

COLDS
Vitamin C
Pantothenic acid
Vitamin P

COLITIS
Iron
Vitamin E

CONSTIPATION
Choline

CYSTITIS
Pantothenic acid
B Complex

DANDRUFF
Vitamin A

DEHYDRATION
Sodium

DEPRESSION
Biotin
Magnesium

DERMATITIS
Biotin

DETACHED RETINA
Vitamin E

DIABETES
Potassium
Zinc
Manganese
Chromatin

DIARRHEA
Folic Acid

DIGESTIVE DISORDERS
Pantothenic acid
Vitamin B2

DISC TROUBLES
Sulphur
Calcium

DIZZINESS
Choline
Manganese
Iron
Vitamin P

DRY SKIN
Paba

ECZEMA
Vitamin B6
Biotin
Vitamin P

EMHYSEMA
Pangamic acid

ENCEPHALITIS
  Vitamin C

FATIGUE
  Folic acid
  Zinc
  Manganese
  Iron

FEVER
  Sodium

FROSTBITE
  Vitamin E

GALLSTONES
  Vitamin A
  Vitamin E

GOITER
  Iodine

GRAY HAIR
  Paba

HAIR COLOR RESTORED
  Paba

HALITOSIS
  Niacin

HAY FEVER
  Vitamin C

HEADACHE
  Choline
  Pangamic acid

HEART DISEASE
Pangamic acid
Inositol
Magnesium
Vitamin E

HEATSTROKE
Sodium

HEMORRHAGE
Vitamin K

HEMORRHOIDS
Vitamin P

HERNIA
Vitamin E

INSOMNIA
Pangamic acid
Choline
Iron
Calcium

JOINT TROUBLES
Sulphur

KIDNEY INFECTION
Vitamin C

KIDNEY STONES
Magnesium

LEG CRAMPS
Niacin
Biotin
Calcium

LIVER PROBLEMS
Vitamin A

LOSS OF TASTE
Zinc

MENINGITIS
Vitamin C

MENOPAUSE
Calcium

MENSTRUAL CRAMPS
Calcium
Vitamin E

MENSTRUAL PROBLEMS
B Complex
Iron
Vitamin K

MENTAL ILLNESS
Folic acid

MENTAL RETARDATION
Vitamin B6

MIGRAINE HEADACHES
Niacin
Vitamin B Complex

MISCARRIAGE
Vitamin P
Vitamin E

MOTION SICKNESS
Vitamin B6

MOUTH SORES
Vitamin B2
Pantothenic acid
Vitamin B6

MUSCULAR DISORDERS
Vitamin B6
Manganese

NAUSEA
Vitamin B1

NERVOUSNESS
Vitamin B6
Iodine

NEURALGIA
Vitamin B1

NIGHT VERSION
Vitamin A

OVERACTIVE THYROID
Iodine
Vitamin E
Paba

OVERWEIGHT
Inositol
B Complex
Vitamin B6
Magnesium
Iodine
Calcium
Vitamin F

PAIN
Vitamin B1
Calcium

PARASITIC DISEASE
Paba

PHLEBITIS
Vitamin C

POISON OAK OR IVY
Vitamin C

Deficiencies and Diseases

POISONOUS BITES
Vitamin C

POLIO
Vitamin C

POOR CIRCULATION
Pangamic acid

PREMATURE AGING
Pangamic acid
Calcium

PROSTATE TROUBLES
Zinc
Magnesium

PSORIASIS
Vitamin F

PSYCHOSIS
B Complex

RADIATION POISON
Vitamin C

RESPIRATORY FLU
Vitamin C
Pantothenic acid

RETARDED GROWTH
Phosphorus
Zinc

RHEUMATIC FEVER
Paba
Vitamin P

RHEUMATISM
Pangamic acid
Vitamin P
Vitamin F
Calcium

ROCKY MTN. SPOTTED FEVER
Paba

SCIATICA
Vitamin B

SENILITY
Niacin

SENSITIVITY TO LIGHT OR SUN
Vitamin B

SHORTNESS OF BREATH
Pangamic acid
Iron

SINUSITIS
Vitamin C
Pantothenic acid
Vitamin E

SKIN SPOTS
Paba

SLIGHT PARALYSIS
Vitamin B

SORETHROAT, STREP
Vitamin C

STERILITY
Zinc
Paba

STOMACH ULCERS
Folic acid
Vitamin P

STRESS
Vitamin C
Paba
Pantothenic acid
Folica cid
B Complex
Phosphorus
Vitamin B6

SUNBURN
Paba

SWOLLEN GLANDS
Vitamin C

TOOTH DECAY
Pantothenic acid
Niacin
Phosphorus
Magnesium
Calcium

ULCERS
Vitamin P
Vitamin E

VIRUS DISEASES
Vitamin C

VOICE BOX GIVES OUT EASILY
Sulphur

WRINKLES
Vitamin A
Vitamin E

With twenty-five 500 milligram tablets, liquified with one-eight cup warm water each teaspoon will equal 1,000 mg; add honey to taste.

Polio virus has been stopped in 72 hours with Vitamin C therapy. We have too long starved the diabetic of fruit sugars and accompanying Vitamin C which would stop the inflammation and running ulcers that seem to go with later stages of diabetes.